IAN OLIO

WHY DO WE DREAM?

MAKE YOUR KID SMART SERIES

For Kids
Ages 4 -9

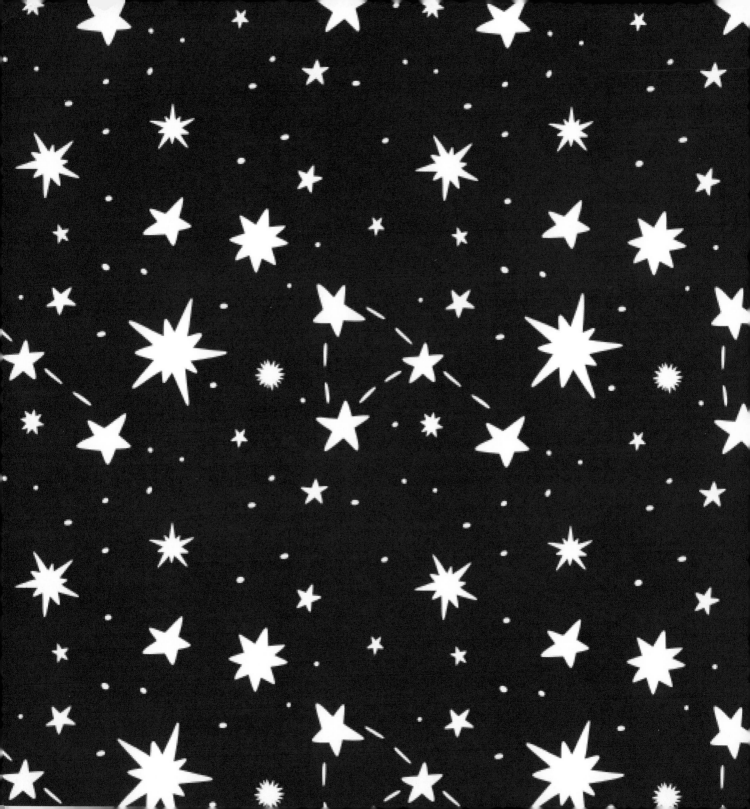

This book belongs to:

....

....

Have you ever wondered
why do we dream?
Or where do our dreams come from?

Scientists think that we have dreams
for a reason.

When we go to sleep, it can look like our bodies and brains are turning off.

But while your body is resting and recharg-ing, your brain actually doesn't rest.

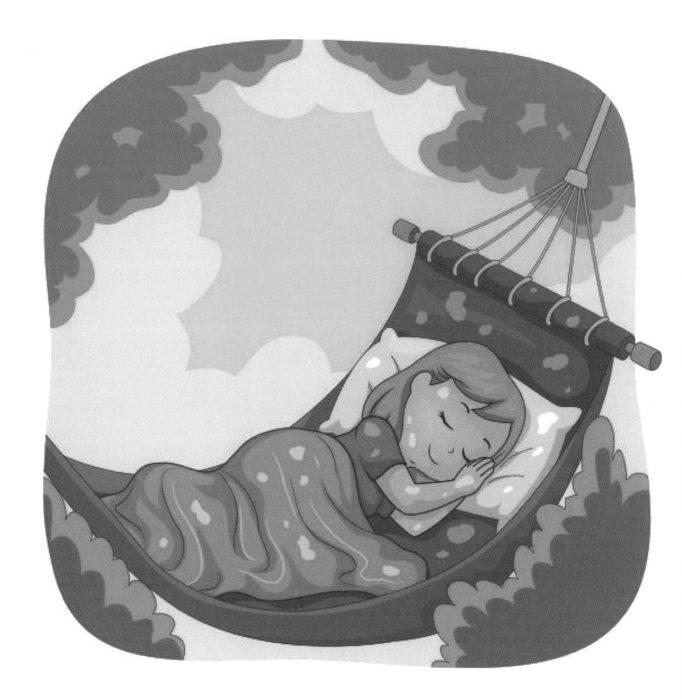

Your brain is working very hard at night releasing all kinds of hormones and chemicals to your body that help you grow.

When you're sleeping, some parts of your brain are switched on, like for example the parts that focus on your feelings.

Your brain is going through different steps of sleep at night. At first you sleep lightly, then your sleep is a bit deeper and you might have a few dreams.

But most of the dreams happen druing the REM sleep. The Rapid Eye Movement stage is the deepest stage of sleep.

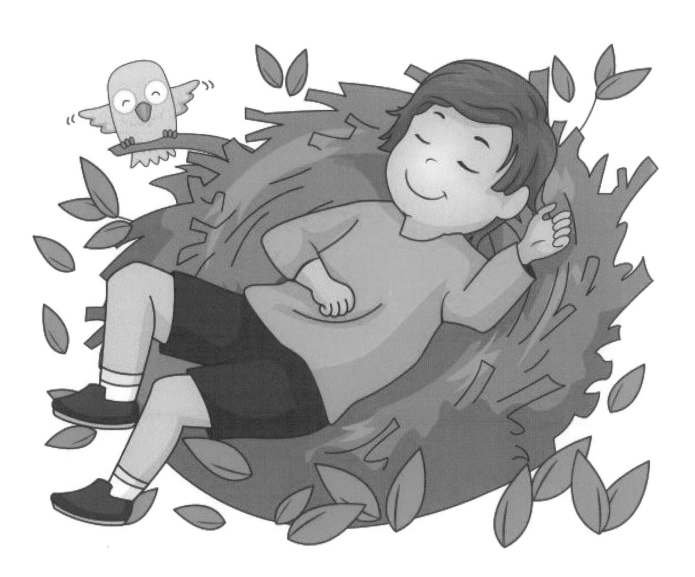

So, why do we dream? Scientists have tried to find an answer to this question for hundreds of thousands of years.

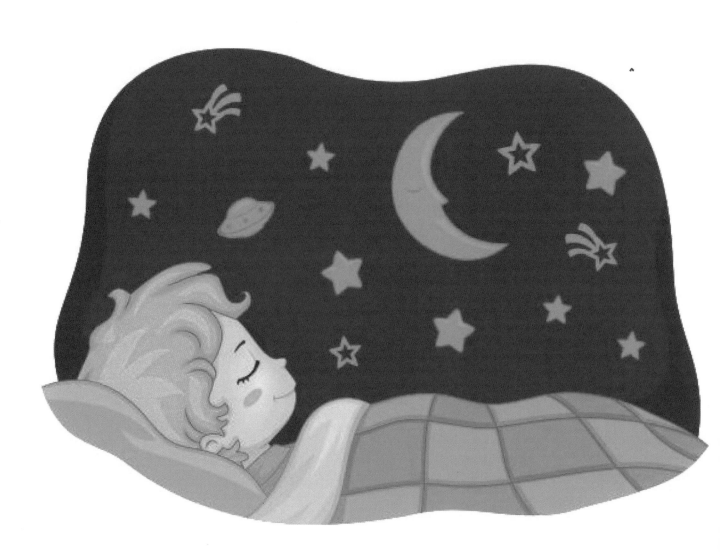

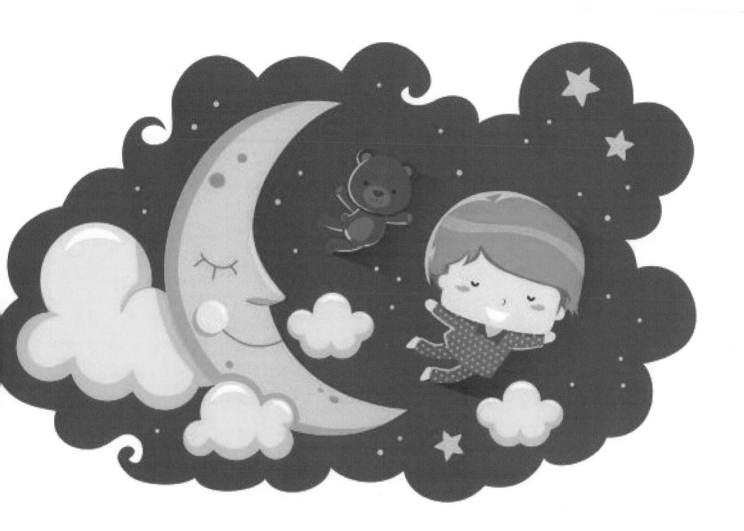

It may surprise you, but despite
the advancements in technology, experts
have not found out yet why people dream.

During the day, you see, hear, smell and experience million of little details about the world around you.

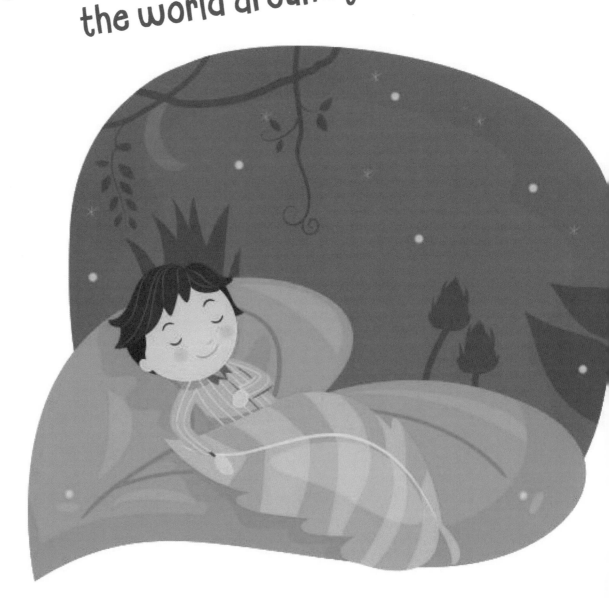

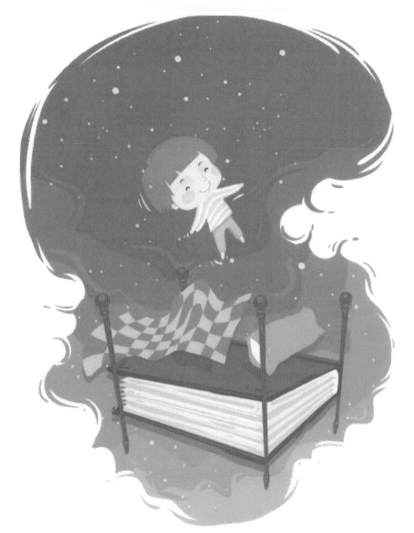

And during the night, your brain needs to store the most important things you've experienced, so that you can remember them for years.

Some scientists think that's what dreams are for, they help you remember the most important things you learned during the day.

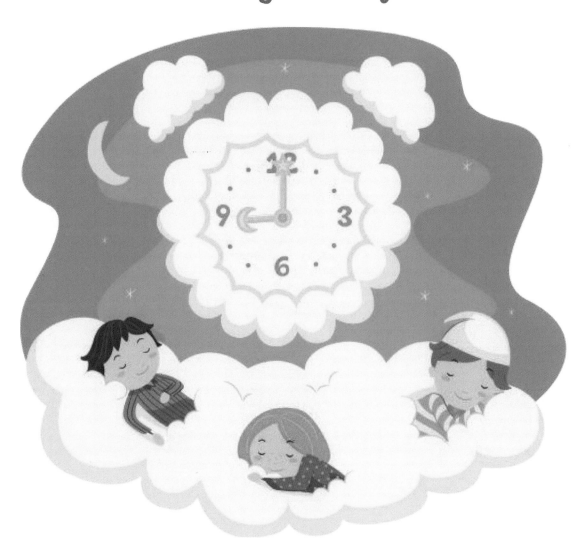

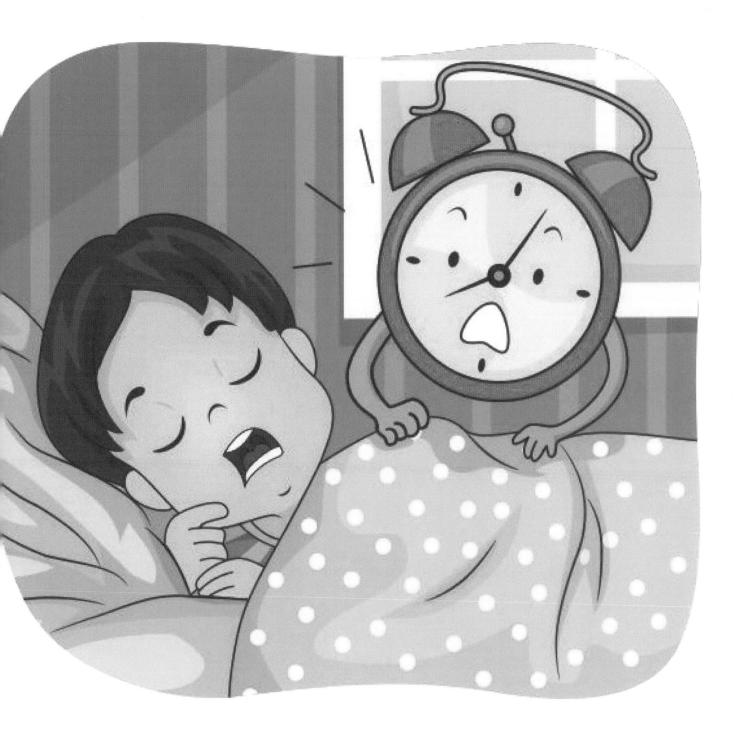

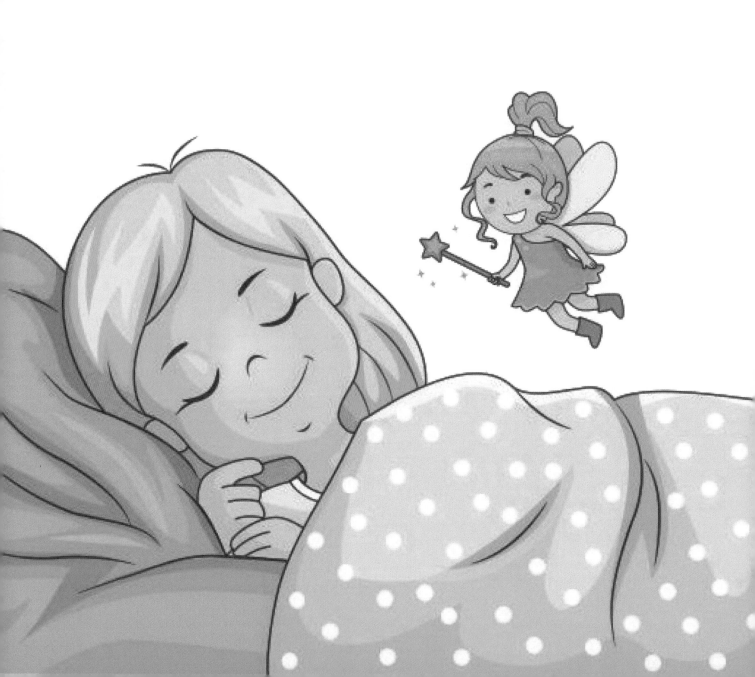

Dreams also help sort out the emotions and feelings you've had throughout the day, so that you are prepared to deal with scary things in the morning.

Dreams play a vital role in our physical, mental and emotional health.

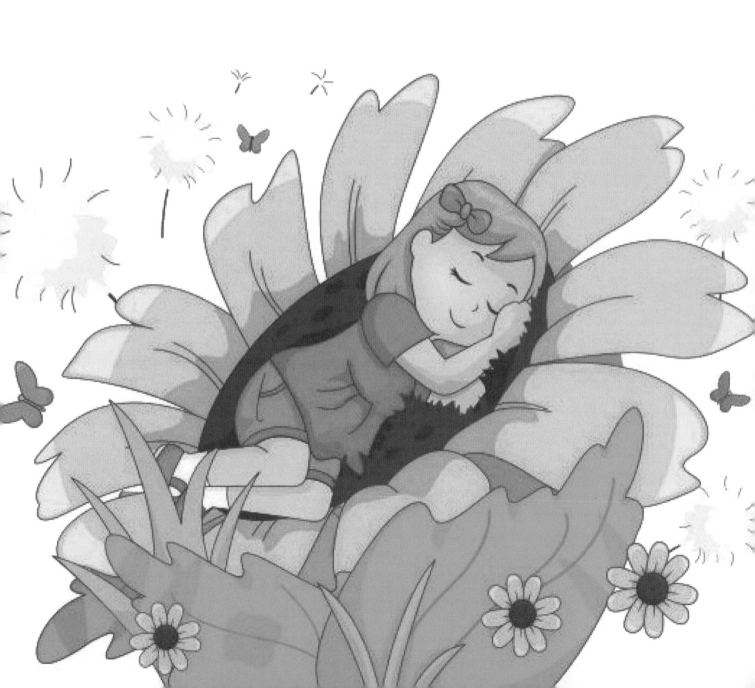

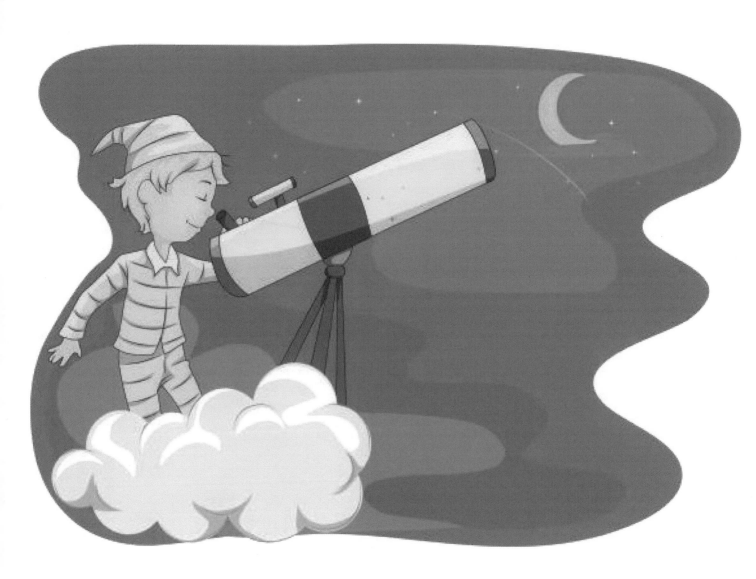

Did you know that most humans sleep approximately 122 days out of every year? That's a lot!

Everybody has dreams at night.
Even if you don't remember your dreams
in the morning, you still have them!

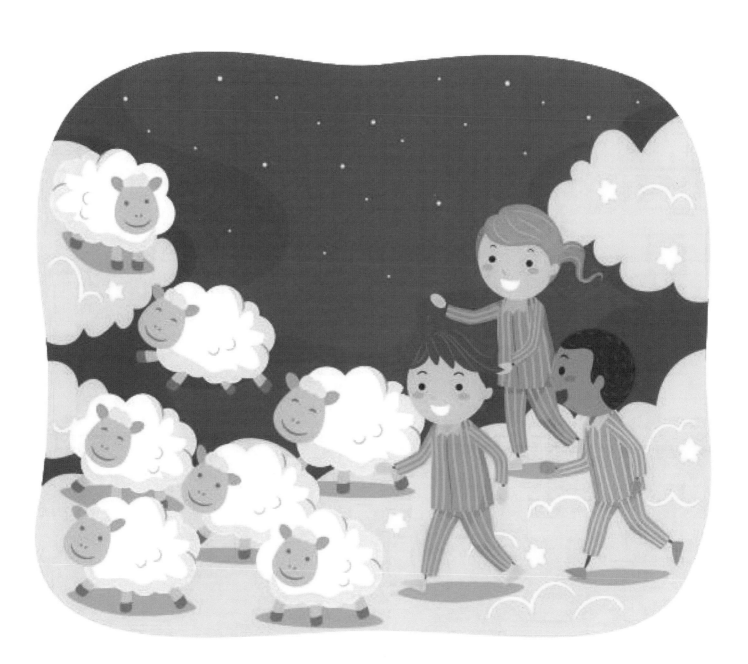

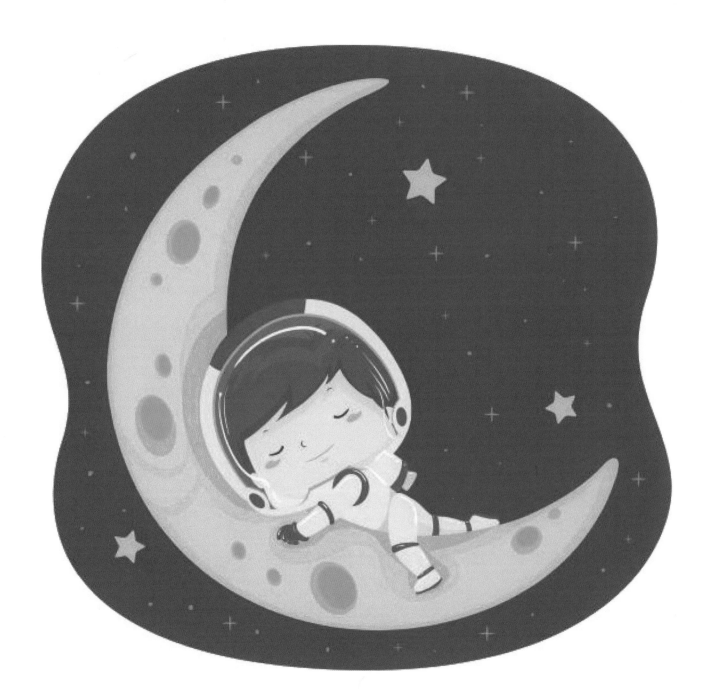

Everybody has dreams at night.
Even if you don't remember your dreams
in the morning, you still have them!

Some animals have dreams too!
It is confirmed that all mammals
experience REM sleep.

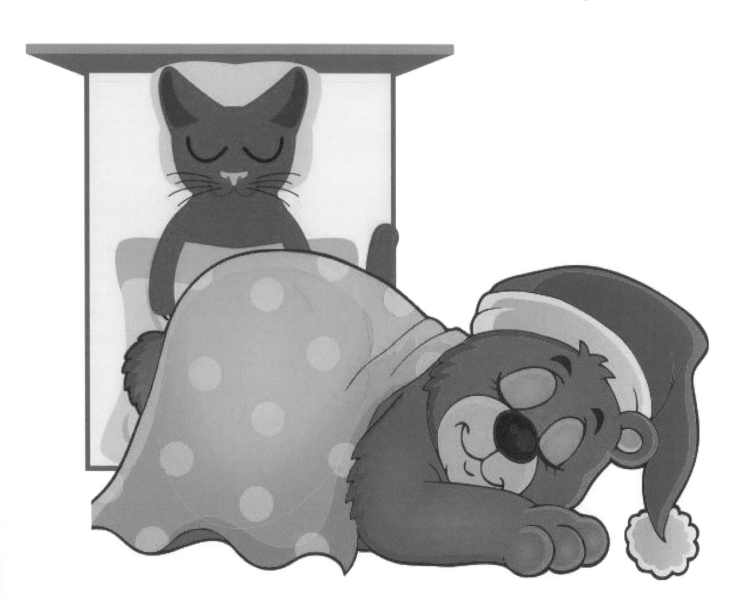

So, animals like
dogs, cats, rats have dreams!
And so do some birds!

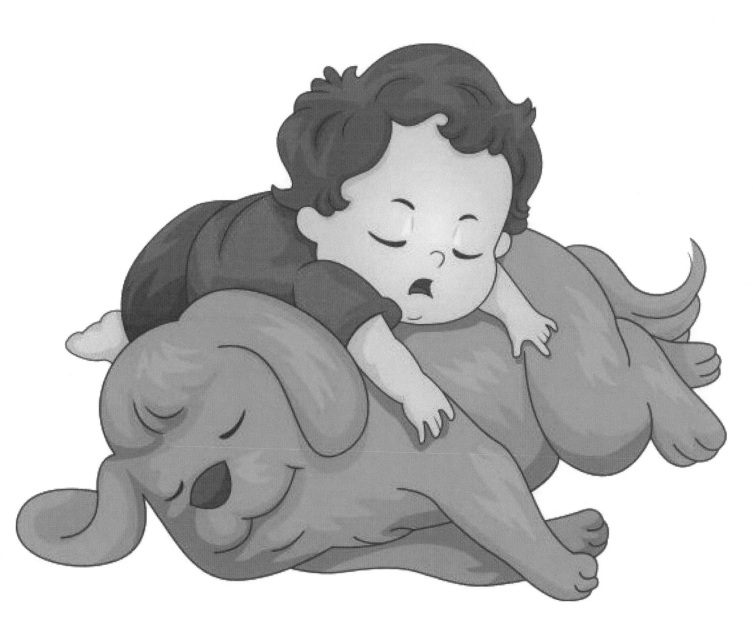

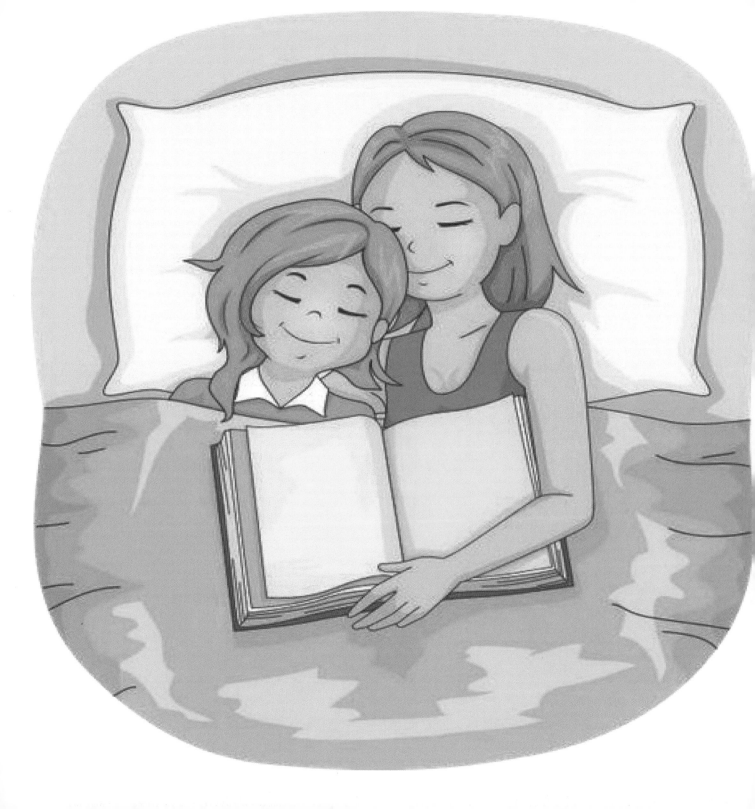

What's the weirdest dream you've ever had?
See you next time friend!

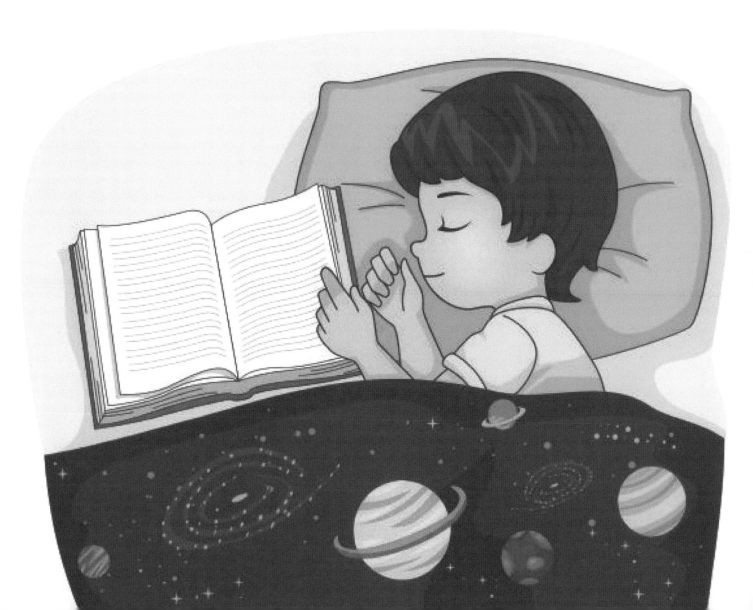

Printed in Great Britain
by Amazon